D1454795

Aural
Rehabilitation

THOMAS G. GIOLAS

5341 Industrial Oaks Boulevard
Austin, Texas 78735

**The PRO-ED
studies in
communicative disorders**

Series editor
HARVEY HALPERN

Library of Congress Cataloging-in-Publication Data
Giolas, Thomas G.
  Aural rehabilitation.

  (The Pro-Ed studies in communicative disorders)
  Includes bibliographies.
  1. Hearing disorders.   2. Hearing disorders—Patients
—Rehabilitation.   I. Title.   II. Series. [DNLM:
1. Hearing Disorders—in adulthood.   2. Hearing
Disorders—rehabilitation. WV 270 G496a]
RF290.G56   1986   617.8'9   86-9375
ISBN 0-89079-097-3

5341 Industrial Oaks Boulevard
Austin, Texas 78735

10 9 8 7 6 5 4 3 2 1   86 87 88 89 90 91

Contents

Preface   v

Introduction   1

Adjustment to Hearing Impairment   5

Problems Associated with the Auditory Mechanism   12

Environmental Conditions   16

Approaches to Aural Rehabilitation   22

Public Information Programs (Prevention)   23

Evaluation   24

Remediation and Reevaluation   25

The Elderly   36

The Educational Setting   36

Summary   38

References   39

Preface

The purpose of this monograph is to introduce the reader to the rehabilitative needs of the hearing-impaired adult. The major emphasis will be on the person who has acquired a hearing impairment after becoming an adult. These persons experience varying degrees of communication problems that adversely affect their social, occupational, and emotional lives. The book discusses these problems as a function of the age at which the hearing impairment occurs, the extent of the hearing loss and its physiological basis, and unfavorable environmental (listening) conditions and communication dynamics. The configuration of these factors, as well as the weighting of each, will vary from person to person. The components of a comprehensive aural rehabilitation program designed to help these individuals are also discussed.

Aural Rehabilitation

Introduction

The last decade has seen an increased emphasis on rehabilitative programs for adults with a hearing impairment. These programs have changed considerably from the lipreading classes of the early years, which centered almost exclusively on improving the hearing-impaired person's ability to obtain meaningful information about what was being said by attending to the visual shape and movement of the speaker's lips (articulators) (O'Neill & Oyer, 1961). Today's aural rehabilitation programs take a broader perspective and look at the overall handicapping effect of hearing impairment. These programs center on communication and the manner in which this process has been disrupted for any given individual. Good verbal communication skills not only facilitate smoother emotional, educational, and social growth, but comprise the main component of the skills necessary for coping with the adult world. Shostrom (1967) believes that communication is the greatest problem human beings face. People spend a great deal of their adult lives attempting to make others understand what they are saying or trying to understand what is being said to them (Fleming, 1972).

The normal development of verbal communication skills depends to a large extent upon the ear's ability to receive and process acoustic energy, especially that which comprises the speech spectrum. Consequently, problems with the normal acquisition of language, speech, education, and vocational skills arise when hearing is impaired. For adults, difficulties become acute in the areas of social interaction and performance in the employment setting, and often considerable strain is placed on interpersonal relationships.

1

The nature and severity of these problems depends on a number of factors, such as (1) the amount of auditory deprivation (hearing loss), (2) the location of the damage in the auditory pathway (site of lesion), and (3) the person's age when the damage occurred (onset of impairment). Other factors include (4) the person's acceptance of the hearing impairment, (5) promptness in seeking professional assistance, (6) family support, and (7) the person's general approach to problem-solving. These latter factors become extremely important in determining the adjustment pattern of a person with a hearing impairment.

This monograph focuses on the effects of hearing impairment in adults and the aural rehabilitative process. Most of the issues discussed here will pertain to persons who have acquired their hearing impairment in adulthood. This is the largest group of adults with a hearing impairment and for whom the majority of aural rehabilitation programs are designed. The needs of the congenitally deaf adult are quite different and beyond the scope of this presentation. There are exceptions, of course, and these exceptions will be discussed in a later section.

Incidence of Hearing Impairment

Approximately 8% of the civilian noninstitutionalized population of the United States report having some degree of difficulty in hearing or understanding speech, including 1% who are deaf (Punch, 1983). Punch reports that this estimate agrees with the recent total estimate of 17.4 million people who are hearing-impaired that was made by the National Center for Health Statistics (1982). Fein (1983) projected that, for the years between 1980 and 2050, the numbers of persons with hearing impairment will increase at a faster rate (102%) than the total U.S. population (36%) as a direct result of aging.

A significant proportion of the hearing-impaired population will be persons who have acquired this impairment after reaching adulthood, and the overall number of hearing-impaired persons grows as a function of age. Figures 1 and 2 illustrate this phenomenon in terms of mean audiometric thresholds for men and women as a function of age. Fein (1983) also points out that while the percentage of hearing-impaired persons aged 65 or over was 43% in 1980, it is projected that the percentage of hearing-impaired persons in this age group will grow to 59% by 2050.

Definition of Terms

The terms *hearing impairment* and *hearing handicap* will have very different meanings when used here. *Hearing impairment* will be used as a generic term referring to any organic hearing problem regardless of etiology or degree. It

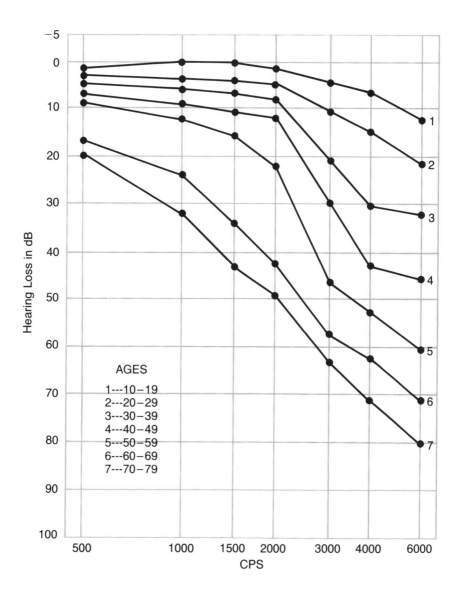

Figure 1. Median hearing losses for men in the total sample of the Wisconsin State Fair Survey. Data are referenced to ASA, 1951, audiometric zero, left ear only. From Glorig et al. (1957, p. 28). Reprinted by permission.

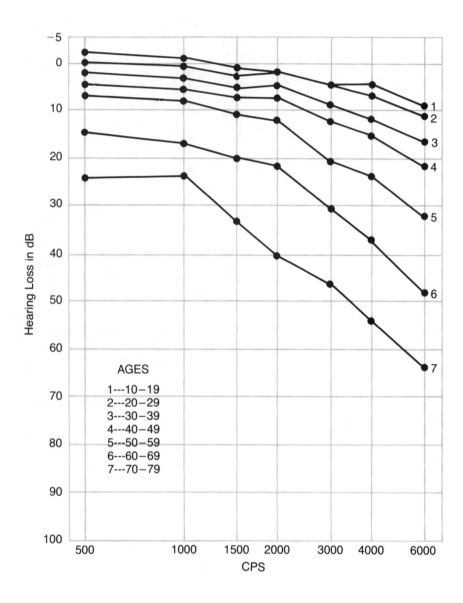

Figure 2.   Median hearing losses for women in the total sample of the Wisconsin State Fair Survey. Data are referenced to ASA, 1951, audiometric zero. From Glorig et al. (1957, p. 29). Reprinted by permission.

will reflect the definition of Davis and Silverman (1978) as "a deviation or change for the worse in either structure or function, usually outside the range of normal" (p. 276). In other words, hearing impairment refers only to the condition of abnormal hearing. *Hearing handicap* refers to the effect of the hearing impairment on the person's everyday situation, or, more specifically, "the disadvantages imposed by an impairment sufficient to affect one's personal efficiency in the activities of daily living" (Davis & Silverman, 1978, p. 276). Aural rehabilitation, therefore, is the process by which the communication disorder specialist assists in reducing the hearing handicap resulting from the hearing impairment.

Two other terms, *hearing loss* and *deaf,* require definition. *Hearing loss* is used whenever a hearing impairment is of a particular magnitude, such as 40 dB. At times *hearing level* will be used interchangeably with *hearing loss.* The term *deaf* will refer to persons in whom the sense of hearing is nonfunctional, with or without amplification, for the ordinary purposes of life. Such an individual may have been born either totally deaf or sufficiently deaf to prevent the establishment of speech and natural language; have become deaf in childhood before language and speech were completely established (prelingual); or have become deaf after having acquired speech and language skills (postlingual), thus significantly impairing communication skills (Nicolosi, Harryman, & Kresheck, 1978). The group of hearing-impaired persons comprising the third category represent the only group of persons for whom the aural rehabilitation programs described in this monograph apply.

It is assumed that the reader has a background in elementary clinical audiology. Basic knowledge is assumed in the following areas: (1) elementary physics of sound, (2) anatomy and physiolgy of the ear, (3) basic ear pathology and treatment, and (4) standard pure-tone and speech audiometric procedures.

Adjustment to Hearing Impairment

For the majority of persons acquiring a hearing impairment as an adult, the process is gradual. Prior to the onset of the hearing impairment, these persons were able to rely on their hearing to assist them in conducting most of their interpersonal, social, and business affairs. They were accustomed to functioning in a hearing world where people spoke to them, they heard and understood what was said, and all was well. They never even had to think about their hearing; it functioned automatically. They did not even have to turn it on, as with vision, in that the eyes must be opened in order to see. Most importantly, they thought of themselves a normally hearing person. It is the natural resistance to changing this self-concept that must be overcome in the initial stages of learning to cope with a hearing impairment.

Slowly, these persons with a gradually acquired hearing impairment become increasingly aware of not always hearing or understanding what has been said. Furthermore, they come to notice that this hearing difficulty occurs even when the room is fairly quiet and devoid of background noises (music, traffic, people talking, etc.). At first, they are convinced they are having difficulty hearing because the speaker is not speaking clearly. They even check this assumption out with a friend who is listening to the same speaker. The friend, who is often close in age and also probably experiencing some hearing difficulty, confirms that the speaker is "mumbling." Even when the person suspects a hearing impairment, there is a tendency to put the blame for the hearing problem on the speaker and not the listener. The situation is further complicated because hearing and understanding are dependent on not only a clear speaker, but also a number of other listening conditions, including room acoustics, paying attention, and good visual cues. These conditions vary sufficiently from listening situation to listening situation so as to thoroughly confuse the person for quite a while. The person does not know whether the auditory failure is a result of a hearing difficulty or one or more of these listening conditions.

However, over time (sometimes years) the number of instances in which the person misinterprets what was said and the number of inappropriate responses increases. These instances are embarrassing, frustrating, and sometimes downright degrading. At the same time, friends and family members are continually suggesting that the person has a hearing problem. The person begins to realize that he or she is not hearing well and that a new approach to handling many everyday affairs must be developed. In other words, the reality of having a hearing impairment begins to materialize and the victim suspects that the standard mode of communication (one that assumes normal hearing) no longer works as well. This realization is very disturbing, and accepting it can be quite an adjustment. Noble (1978) believes that the partial loss of hearing in adulthood can be extremely traumatic. He writes, "No preparation has been made for such a transition, and the solitary nature of the occurrence leaves the individual with a feeling of bereavement" (p. 18).

Once this stage of awareness occurs, the adjustment pattern followed varies from person to person. It is generally agreed that the more severe and sudden the hearing impairment, the more complicated the reaction and adjustment. At the same time, clinical experience suggests that most persons acquiring a hearing impairment as adults will experience some degree of emotional reaction, regardless of the nature and onset of the impairment. Most people go through several stages of adjustment (some of which can go on for most of their lives) in the process of adjusting to and compensating for the handicapping effects of a hearing impairment.

Rousey (1971) writes that the nature of the adjustment pattern is closely related to the way common human emotions, known as *affects,* are inappropriately expressed as a result of a threat to one's well-being and personal integrity. Affects are defined as feelings of love, longing, jealousy, mortification, pain, and mourning as well as feelings of hatred, anger, and rage. Rousey (1971) views hearing impairments as constituting a sufficient threat to "... exacerbate longstanding problems in dealing with affect." In other words, the hearing impairment is seen as a sufficiently serious irritant to trigger a number of behaviors typically used to deal with severe frustration and personal threat.

Hearing-impaired persons must then rely on ingrained internal affects to respond to their environment. If these internal affects are relatively healthy, they will serve these individuals well. However, if they are unstable, the result may be the opposite.

According to Rousey (1971), the major reactions associated with hearing impairment are projection and denial. Rousey defines *projection* as what occurs when "an individual attributes to others in his environment some unpleasant wishes and feelings that he is experiencing within himself" (p. 387). *Denial* is defined by Rousey (1971) as defensive behavior used when one feels severe internal stress or external pressures in situations in which affects are threatening to become uncontrollable. Evidences of the defense mechanism of denial are seen daily in the audiology clinic. There are those who refuse to acknowledge that they need a hearing aid when it is quite clear to the audiologist as well as to the family. There are parents of deaf children who refuse to accept the diagnosis of hearing impairment and will spend many more months, even years, looking for a more favorable diagnosis, wasting precious habilitative years.

Once the defense mechanisms are terminated or temporarily abandoned (or even while they are being used), the hearing-impaired person may experience one or more feelings of affect. Rousey (1971) states that two affects typically associated with hearing impairment are mourning and mortification. Both of these reactions have been observed in the clinical setting in one form or another. One patient who acquired a sudden severe hearing loss in both ears actually spoke of the "death" of her hearing. For a period of time, she went through a mourning experience. A second person displayed the affect of mortification in the form of shame. He was convinced that he would be ostracized or even punished for having a hearing impairment. Rousey (1971) writes that these feelings are often considered derivatives of shame. Still another woman displayed mortification in a more general sense by devoting an inordinate amount of time to wondering why such an awful thing had happened to her.

One of the more observable reactions to hearing loss of differing degrees is the feeling of depression. Ramsdell (1978) attempts to explain these feelings of depression as a function of the way the hearing impairment has interfered with three levels of hearing: (1) the primitive, (2) the signal or warning, and (3) the symbolic.

Primitive Level

While interference with all three of these levels contributes in varying degrees to the depression, interference with the primitive level is often viewed as the most significant. The primitive level of hearing is the way normally hearing people add depth to the world around them. Even though they are mostly unaware of it, they are constantly extending their environment beyond the person with whom they are speaking, and even beyond their sphere of vision, by attending to background sounds that are peculiar to that particular environment. For example, consider the person who is in a lecture hall listening to a speaker. In addition to this conscious, deliberate use of hearing, the person is also attending in a somewhat semiconscious way to a number of environmental background sounds, such as those made by an air conditioner or by people shuffling their feet or coughing randomly. All these background sounds contribute to making the total environment more alive acoustically and more multidimensional. They connect the normally hearing person with the world much more fully than the conscious, deliberate level of hearing does by itself.

When hearing impairment becomes sufficiently extensive to interfere with or diminish the ability to hear the auditory background noises of daily living, confusion and depression often occur, and the hearing-impaired person may experience the world as dead. One person who had acquired a sudden severe bilateral hearing loss reported that the sudden silence gave her the feeling that something ominous had happened in the world and that everyone was mourning a death. Ramsdell (1978) describes the effect of hearing loss at the primitive level as follows: "It [the primitive level] relates us to the world at a very primitive level, somewhere below the level of clear consciousness and perception. The loss of this feeling or relationship with the world is the major cause of the well-recognized feeling of 'deafness,' and also of the depression that permeates the suddenly deafened and, to a lesser degree, those in whom deafness develops gradually" (p. 501).

As changes in the environmental sounds occur and are responded to, a new phenomenon emerges. The normally hearing person is no longer only hearing these sounds on the primitive level, but has moved on to a more conscious level of hearing. In the example used earlier, the person listening on a semiconscious level (the primitive level) to the air conditioner uses that sound as one parameter to define the environment, and when the air conditioner stops because the room has reached the desired temperature, the person quickly notices that the room acoustics have changed and are now minus that sound. If one multiplies that event by a number of such auditory changes that are occurring in one's auditory world, one can begin to see that normal hearing provides the feeling that the room is not only alive but ever-changing. It is this phenomenon of a changing world that provides the person with a sense of security and a readiness for immediate changes. For many hearing-impaired persons, the loss of the auditory cues that indicate these changes is particularly annoying, especially because they do not quite understand what has taken place.

In summary, the primitive level of hearing provides a very important and basic contribution to a person's general feeling of security. It is the basic ingredient which creates a background of feeling, which Ramsdell (1978) calls *affective tone* (p. 501). In the semiconscious listening stage it connects people with their immediate auditory environment, helping them to feel a part of a living active world. As they become aware of the auditory background of their daily living, they are attuned to changes occurring in it and are in a state of readiness to react appropriately. Interference with this level of hearing causes a number of problems, which will be discussed in more detail in a later section.

Signal or Warning Level

The second level of hearing, called the *signal* or *warning,* consists of a more conscious level of listening that provides people with valuable information about what is going on in the world around them. Normally hearing persons are constantly aware of sounds within their hearing range. For example, they are often aware of what is going on in other rooms of the house, whether someone is walking around upstairs or coming down the stairs, when someone comes into the room (even if that person is out of their line of vision), which direction a sound is coming from, whether someone in another car is blowing a horn at them, and a host of other auditory events. These signals serve as warnings and allow normally hearing persons to react appropriately. For example, when they hear the siren of an ambulance or police car, they typically slow down and pull over to the right side of the street. Failure to do so can certainly be embarassing, if not dangerous. The security afforded normally hearing persons as a result of their ability to hear most sounds within their range of hearing as well as to identify the direction of a sound must not be underestimated.

Symbolic Level

The highest and most refined level of hearing is that level which allows people to organize auditory events into meaningful language units or symbols. These symbols are used to communicate verbally with others. Ramsdell (1978) calls this level the *symbolic level.* The symbolic level requires the best hearing acuity of the three levels described, and interference with this level causes a host of communication problems. These problems and the conditions under which they occur will be the topic of the next section.

Regardless of the particular adjustment pattern a hearing-impaired person experiences, Shontz's (1967) theoretical model of dealing with a crisis is quite helpful in understanding the complexity of the adjustment. Shontz discusses *crisis* as the result of an event which causes "... a sudden requirement to restructure psychological organization" (p. 364). He describes five phases, each of which, when applied to the process of adjusting to an acquired hearing impairment, has some interesting implications.

Shock

The first phase outlined by Shontz is that of *shock* and represents the initial encounter with the critical situation. This phase might be thought of as the point when the hearing-impaired person is told, most often by a professional, that a hearing impairment does indeed exist, and that it is of sufficient magnitude to require remedial help, even a hearing aid. Furthermore, no medical treatment can alleviate the problem. The impact of this news is often greater than is assumed. This is when the person's worst fears are confirmed. Shontz (1967) describes this phase as encompassing feelings of numbness, as if there was no feeling or no self. During this phase, it is apparent that little information (e.g., extent of loss, type of hearing disorder, remediation plans, etc.) is being processed. This phase may shed light on why clinicians often have to repeat everything to a patient that was said during the initial audiological visit. It should also motivate clinicians to consider going somewhat slower in the initial stages of reporting hearing test results.

Realization

Shock is followed by a *realization* or awareness of the condition. This awareness can produce fear and panic that still prevent persons from perceiving their condition accurately. The person can appear highly anxious and overwhelmed by the whole situation. While realization is an important phase, it does not mean the person has understood or accepted the hearing impairment. The person may be aware of the existence of the hearing problem but still deny its seriousness. When a person is in this phase, too much remedial planning may not be productive.

Defensive Retreat

The third phase is called *defensive retreat*. Persons in this phase would like to retreat to a precondition (normal hearing) state. They would like to act as if the hearing impairment did not happen. Some refer to this behavior as denial, repression, or suppression. This phase often explains why patients resist amplification suggestions, seek a second opinion, or fail to keep follow-up appointments.

Acknowledgment

Acknowledgment can follow the phase of retreat. This phase differs from the realization phase in that, in spite of continued concern and anxiety, the person is ready to start doing something about the problem. The person becomes much more receptive to remediation suggestions. Although these suggestions often bring on new forms of stress and anxiety, this is the point at which the remediation program takes a big step in a positive direction and the person is eager to cooperate. It is the phase to be reached before performing a hearing aid evaluation.

Adaptation

The final phase is *adaptation* and is viewed as the period of adjustment, which implies change. Shontz (1967) describes this phase as consisting of a reintegration of self, a renewed sense of worth, an attitude quite different from the old sense of well-being (i.e., "I've been through the crisis and I feel that I understand these things better now"). He suggests that "major changes are adaptive in nature, and the watchwords are 'setbacks' and 'successes' " (p. 7). The former impose themselves, and the latter seem to come with painful slowness. Anyone who has conducted an aural rehabilitation group recognizes this phase in those persons who have made great strides in learning to compensate for their hearing impairment but who at the same time express repeated frustration with the number of listening situations that continue to be bothersome and out of their control.

In conclusion, it is important to emphasize that the process of adjusting to the day-to-day reality of a hearing impairment is a complex one. While several options and models have been presented, they are just that—options and models. Very little research has been conducted to map the most common or preferred approach to adjustment. This is probably so because hearing impairments and those who have them come packaged in many different ways. As a result, it is very difficult to predict the adjustment pattern a given individual will follow or even to prescribe a preferred pattern. As a result, clinicians should maintain an open mind, be good listeners, and take their lead from the affected person when planning the rehabilitative program.

Problems Associated with the Auditory Mechanism

The problems typically associated with a hearing impairment acquired in adulthood result from a deterioration of the auditory processing mechanism and its effect on the reception and interpretation of the speech code. These problems can be grouped under three general headings: (1) the effect of reduced audibility, (2) the effect of reduced speech discrimination ability, and (3) the contribution of environmental conditions to overall communication effectiveness. The discussion of these conditions will center on the associated communication problems.

Reduced Audibility

One of the common symptoms of a hearing impairment is reduced audibility of speech and other auditory signals. That is, more intensity is necessary to produce an awareness of stimulation or threshold (Nicolosi, Harryman, & Kreshek, 1978) for the hearing-impaired person. Consequently, it is more difficult to hear and understand what is being said in most normal listening situations. For purposes of this discussion, *hearing* is defined as being aware of an auditory signal, and *understanding* is defined as hearing the words the other person is saying clearly enough to be able to participate in the conversation. For example, it is generally accepted that conversational speech is heard at approximately 45 dB HL (ANSI, 1969). A person who has an audiometrically measured hearing level of 45 dB would receive normal conversational speech quite faintly, miss faint speech altogether, and receive loud speech at a comfortable level. This example assumes a quiet listening situation. Noisy settings would make the listening task even more difficult. The hearing-impaired person would have considerable difficulty in many talking, learning, and working situations.

When one takes into account the wide range of intensity covered by speech sounds, the problem is further complicated. Individual speech phonemes vary, depending on how they are measured, by as much as 30 to 35 dB. This is further complicated by the fact that conversational speech is a dynamic process in which the intensity range of the message alters from moment to moment depending on the talker's speaking volume, stress patterns, and distance from the listener.

In conclusion, the nature of the alteration of speech with respect to intensity are functions of an interaction between the acoustic parameters of individual phonemes, the conversational context (prosodic features) in which they occur, and the hearing impairment of the listener. The primary behavioral symptom of persons with a conductive hearing disorder is reduced audibility, resulting from reduced efficiency of the middle ear.

Reduced Speech Discrimination

One of the more common problems of persons with hearing impairment is the lack of clarity in the speech they hear. Depending on the nature of the impairment, speech will be distorted to some degree. Audiologists are often told, "Speech is loud enough for me; it's just not clear enough," or "Now that I'm wearing my hearing aid, I can hear people; I just can't understand what they are saying." Speech discrimination is generally measured clinically by presenting hearing-impaired persons with a speech message at predetermined levels above their threshold and obtaining a measure of how well they were able to repeat what was said. It is assumed that there is a close relationship between the ability to repeat the speech message presented and the level of difficulty that is experienced in most conversational situations. While there are a number of other factors contributing to a person's communicative efficiency, the degree to which the speech signal is received clearly plays a major role.

A number of studies have been conducted dealing with the adult's ability to identify various components of the speech signal under a number of acoustic conditions. The general concern of these studies is aimed at gaining some insight into what the spoken message sounds like to hearing-impaired persons — which speech categories are interfered with as a result of their auditory configuration and which categories are more available to them. While the results of these studies do not wholly agree on all aspects of speech discrimination among the hearing-impaired, it is generally accepted that persons with acquired hearing impairments experience less difficulty identifying vowels than consonants regardless of their audiometric configuration. More specifically findings with regard to vowel and consonent discrimination include:

1. Persons with hearing impairments that have been corrected by amplification do not have serious discrimination problems with vowels.
2. Such persons experience varying degrees of difficulty with consonants, depending upon the audiometric configuration.
3. There is no systematic set of error responses associated with etiology.
4. Normally hearing persons listening to distorted speech produce error responses quite similar to those of hearing-impaired persons. This finding

is most helpful to the clinician who wishes to generalize from data obtained with normally hearing persons and apply it to hearing-impaired persons who have grown up with normal hearing. Both populations have the benefit of acoustic, linguistic, and environmental redundancy and find themselves in a position where this redundancy is slowly diminishing.

5. Hearing above 2000 Hz plays an extremely important role in speech discrimination.

For a more thorough understanding of these and other pertinent findings, consult the research of Owens et al. (1968a, 1968b, 1972, 1980).

Special Types of Hearing Impairment

Persons with a *unilateral hearing impairment* demonstrate a number of communication problems specific to monaural hearing. Giolas and Wark (1967) interviewed 20 persons with unilateral hearing impairments. The interviews were designed to define the specific situations in which a monaurally hearing person has difficulty communicating. Secondary considerations dealt with the actions taken in response to each situation reported and the feelings associated with these situations. The critical-incident technique (Flanagan, 1954) was employed. Table 1 lists the categories which emerged from the incidents reported.

The feelings associated with various listening situations, as well as general statements made during the course of the interviews, suggested that these individuals experienced considerably more communication difficulty than may have been assumed in the past. The majority expressed such negative feelings as embarrassment, annoyance, confusion, and helplessness. These negative feelings occurred most often in situations where those present were unaware of the individual's hearing impairment.

Another type of hearing impairment is *presbycusis,* a gradual loss of hearing that is one of the common results of aging. Presbycusis is seen as a combination of the many physical parameters (including altered hearing) associated with the aging process as well as the psychological, environmental, and behavioral manifestations of this process.

One of the more obvious clinical characteristics of presbycusis is a reduction in sensitivity to pure tones. Figures 1 and 2 plot the median hearing losses for men and women, respectively. It is apparent that there is a steady loss of sensitivity to pure tones, especially in the higher frequencies, as a function of age. This conclusion has been substantiated with surprising consistency over the years by a number of investigators.

A second very common characteristic of presbycusis is poor speech discrimination. The specific problems comprising this characteristic are similar to

TABLE 1
Communication Problems Reported by Persons with a Unilateral Hearing Loss

Categories	Total Incidents Reported	Number of Persons Contributing to Each Category
Difficulty hearing or understanding speech when it was presented to the impaired ear while the normal ear was partially or fully masked by extraneous noise.	26	16
Difficulty hearing or understanding speech when it was presented to the impaired ear while no appreciable extraneous noise masked the normal ear.	12	9
Difficulty understanding speech when subject was situated in a setting which contained a great deal of extraneous noise, regardless of whether the stimulus was directed toward the good or the bad ear.	12	9
Difficulty understanding speech when subject was situated in a relatively quiet setting, regardless of whether stimulus was directed toward the good or the bad ear.	18	9
Difficulty distinguishing from which direction a given auditory stimulus came in the presence of considerable extraneous noise.	18	11
Difficulty distinguishing from which direction a given auditory stimulus came in a relatively quiet setting.	12	8
Miscellaneous	2	2

Source: Giolas and Wark (1967, p. 338). Reprinted by permission.

those described earlier with one exception. The problem in some elderly persons can appear to be inconsistent with the extent of threshold deficit for pure tones, including those of high frequency. In other words, the reduced responsiveness to verbal messages (and probably nonverbal messages) is more pronounced than what would be expected and typically observed with younger people who have similar audiometric configurations. Hull (1977) describes this phenomenon as consisting of auditory comprehension, cognition, and the sorting of both the phonemic and linguistic features of speech, and he concludes that the cause must be at some level beyond the cochlea and eighth nerve. This phenomenon was first identified by Gaeth (1948), who called it *phonemic regression.*

As there is a general reduction of responsiveness to auditory stimuli as a function of the aging process, it follows that there may also be reduced responsiveness to visual stimuli. Binnie (1973) writes:

> The causes of visual deterioration among the aged may be related to (1) external changes in the eye, (2) alterations in the condition of the lens, and (3) intraocular conditions. Moreover, problems in visual perceptual performance such as reduced visual memory, retention and response time may contribute to the overall reduction in visual and auditory-visual speech comprehension. (p. 135)

While the exact cause of this reduced efficiency is not fully understood, the result is often a decreased potential for the optimal use of visual cues in the communication process.

While the primary nature of the hearing impairment associated with presbycusis is sensorineural, there is some evidence that persons with hearing difficulty as a function of age can demonstrate a conductive component (Glorig, Wheeler, Quiggle, Grings, & Summerfield, 1957). Furthermore, this component, reflected audiometrically as an air-bone gap, appears at the affected higher frequencies. While there is some controversy over the validity of this phenomenon, it does make sense that the general deterioration associated with the aging process would affect all physical structures of the peripheral auditory mechanism.

It is important to remember that we have been talking about group characteristics associated with persons who have presbycusis. The degree to which any one person exhibits any one of the problems described varies tremendously and is dependent on a host of physical, psychological, and environmental factors.

Environmental Conditions

The communication problems associated with a hearing impairment are further exacerbated by environmental conditions. This section will explore the components of environmental noise, communication dynamics, and auditory failure.

Environmental Noise

One of the most common complaints expressed by persons with a sensorineural hearing impairment is that they have considerable difficulty understand-

TABLE 2
Approximate Sound Pressure Levels of Familiar Environmental Sounds

	Decibels	
Jet engine (100 feet)	140	Pain threshold
		Air-raid siren
Riveting gun	130	Threshold of feeling (tickle)
Thunder	120	Turbine generators
Modern discotheque		
	110	Loud shout (1 foot)
Power lawnmower		Diesel truck (high speed)
New York subway	100	Motorcycle (no muffler)
Jackhammer		Electric blender
Shouted speech	90	Speech interference level
		City traffic (inside car)
	80	Loud singing (not amplified)
Noisy restaurant	70	
	60	Normal speaking level
	50	Average office
Quiet residence		
	40	Quiet office
	30	Faint whisper

Source: Lipscomb (1970, p. 2). Reprinted by permission.

ing speech in the presence of background noise. Typical noisy conditions include background music in restaurants, music from hi-fi sets, and music superimposed on TV voice tracks; noises produced by household appliances such as air conditioners, dehumidifiers, dishwashers, and window fans; and the overall noise produced by numbers of people talking simultaneously.

Table 2 lists a number of familiar environmental noises and their decibel levels. Normal conversational speech occurs at approximately 77 dB SPL, so if many of these sounds are present while conversation is attempted, much of the speech message will be rendered unintelligible even if hearing is normal.

Any sound introduced into a room is altered considerably by the acoustic characteristics of the room. These changes, including the intensity ratio between the primary source (speech) and various background sounds, can combine to render conversational speech difficult to understand even for persons with normal hearing. More important, there is considerable evidence that persons with sensorineural hearing impairments experience considerably more difficulty understanding speech in noisy conditions than do persons with normal hearing when listening to speech under identical conditions (Crum & Tillman, 1973; Nabelek & Pickett, 1974a, 1974b; Tillman, Carhart, & Olsen, 1974). The hearing impairment produces reduced intensity as well as altered frequency and temporal characteristics that require more favorable room acoustics for adequate speech intelligibility in the case of the hearing-impaired. A more complete discussion of the deleterious effects of poor room acoustics can be found in Ross (1978).

To complete the discussion regarding difficulty experienced by the hearing-impaired as a function of noise, it should be noted that in some cases amplification can contribute adverse effects. This is a function of the creation of an upward spread of masking that obscures the valuable high frequencies essential to good speech discrimination or the creation of a tolerance problem that if not properly considered will produce unnecessary distortion.

Communication Dynamics

We have been discussing sensorineural hearing impairment in terms of its effect on communication. So far we have considered the following factors: (1) adjustment to the hearing impairment, (2) the frequency, intensity, and time restriction of the spoken message (hearing impairment), (3) personal amplification (the hearing aid), and (4) the physical characteristics of the environment (room acoustics).

In order to complete the picture, a host of additional conditions which comprise the communication process and which have a great influence on the success or failure of a communication event must be discussed. These conditions include (1) the person with whom the speaker is talking (relationship of the speaker to the listener), (2) under what conditions the communicative act is occurring (number of speakers, environmental noise conditions, etc.), (3) the purpose of the verbal intercourse (social, work, business), and (4) the response to the auditory failure. In order to fully appreciate what it means to have a hearing impairment, we must explore the role of these communication dynamics.

One of the most comprehensive studies exploring the social implications of hearing impairment was conducted by Nett, Doerfler, and Matthews (1960). The study was designed to investigate the effects of hearing impairment on the daily life experiences of hearing-impaired adults. A total of 378 hearing-impaired persons were interviewed and tested both audiologically and psychologically. In addition, 246 spouses, friends, relatives, and work associates were inter-

TABLE 3
Number of Critical Incidents Reported in Four Life Areas

Life Area	Number	%
Social	493	43
Family	266	23
Vocational	256	23
Social-Business	124	11
Total	1,139	100

Source: Nett, Doerfler, and Matthews (1960, p. 56). Reprinted by permission.

viewed. The critical-incident interviewing technique (Flanagan, 1954) was used. The results of these interviews offer considerable insight into the communication problems experienced by the hearing-impaired adult.

Table 3 contains a breakdown of the number of critical communication incidents reported in four settings: social, family, vocational, and social-business. (The first three categories are self-explanatory; an example of the social-business category is the situation involving a real estate agent. The agent is in the hearing-impaired person's home in a quasisocial atmosphere, but the purpose of the interaction is purely business.) For those who have worked with hearing-impaired adults who are gradually losing their hearing, it is not surprising that the greatest number of critical incidents reported are in the area of social situations. It is here that they feel the greatest impact on their lifestyle. Table 4 provides a breakdown of the number of incidents reported in each life area by the various respondents.

Table 5 reports the type of problems reported in the life areas. The incidents were broken down primarily into four major categories: (1) those in which no auditory failure actually occurred; (2) those in which there was a failure to hear an auditory stimulus; (3) those in which there was a failure to understand or interpret speech or music; and (4) those in which there was a failure to localize an auditory stimulus. These categories were then broken down into more specific problems. The table shows the frequency with which these difficulties occurred in this group. Approximately 70% of the incidents involved failure to understand speech or music, while only 20% involved failure to hear a stimulus. The fact that so many of the reported incidents centered around the problem of understanding speech reinforces the need for aural rehabilitation programs to concentrate on this area.

There appears to be a consistent relationship between the kind of auditory problem reported and the communicative setting in which it occurs. The sub-

TABLE 4
Number of Critical Incidents per Person Reporting in Each Life Area, by Type of Respondent

Type of Respondent	Life Area			
	Social	Family	Vocational	Business-Social
Patient	1.2	.5	1.0	.3
Spouse	.5	.7	.0	.1
Relative	.5	.4	.0	.1
Friend	.8	.0	.0	.1
Coworker, Employer	.3	.01	1.2	.1

Source: Nett, Doerfler, and Mathews (1960, p. 56). Reprinted by permission.

TABLE 5
Type of Problems Reported in Critical Incidents

Type of Problem	Number		%
Other than auditory failure	80		7
Series of failures implied		78	
Auditory illusion		2	
Failure to hear stimulus	239		21
Signal (bell, buzzer, bark)		80	
Natural speech		151	
Amplified speech or music		8	
Failure to understand speech or music	797		70
Natural speech		709	
Amplified speech		88	
Failure to localize sound	23		2
Total	1139		100

Source: Nett, Doerfler, and Matthews (1960, p. 60). Reprinted by permission.

jects reported that both hearing failures and understanding failures occur most often when the person is in a small informal group of two or more persons. Hearing failures also occur frequently when the person is alone (they are informed later that they missed a phone call, didn't answer the doorbell, etc.), while understanding failures also occur fairly frequently in small or large formal

TABLE 6
Response to Auditory Failure

Reponse	Number	%
Ask for repetition	203	28
Obtain assistance	102	14
Pretend, guess, or bluff	98	14
Intentionally do nothing	89	12
Get into a better position	67	9
Make a mechanical adaptation	56	8
Ask for repetition and get into a better position	28	4
Withdraw	27	4
Tell about loss beforehand	23	3
Depend on sight	17	2
Read lips	11	2
Total	721	100

Source: Nett, Doefler, and Matthews (1960, p. 60). Reprinted by permission.

groups. It is interesting to note that more auditory failures were reported as occurring in informal situations than in formal situations.

An interesting part of this study consisted of asking the hearing-impaired subjects what they did when they experienced an auditory failure. Eleven separate responses, one of which was a combination of two of the other responses, were reported. These are listed in order of frequency of occurrence in Table 6.

The two responses reported most often ("ask for repetition" and "obtain assistance") are excellent rehabilitative actions that suggest good adjustment to the hearing impairment. However, the next two most often reported responses ("pretend, guess, or bluff" and "intentionally do nothing") are certain to cause the hearing-impaired person problems. What is even more disturbing is how few people reported using such appropriate responses as "get into a better position," "make a mechanical adaptation," "ask for repetition and get into a better position," "tell about loss beforehand," and "depend on sight."

The hearing-impaired subjects also reported 290 incidents in which they were unable to respond at all to an auditory failure. What is disturbing is that in 244 of these incidents, the person was not even aware of the auditory failure until later, and consequently was not in a position to correct the situation at the time it occurred. As a result, the subjects later learned they had given incorrect responses to questions, had interrupted conversations, or had talked about subjects different from those under discussion. In the remaining 46 incidents in which the hearing-impaired person did not respond, someone else interceded (that is, answered the question addressed to the person, told someone he or she did not hear and asked for repetition, etc.).

Approaches to Aural Rehabilitation

Aural rehabilitation for hearing-impaired adults is a multifaceted process and unfortunately is often viewed differently by professionals, depending on their orientation and service setting. In the early years, aural rehabilitation was viewed as consisting exclusively of lipreading classes. These early classes were designed to help hearing-impaired persons become more proficient at recognizing individual sounds made on the lips. The rationale was that considerable information about what the speaker is saying can be gleaned from lip movements alone; more will be said about this later. In recent years, these classes were expanded to include the use of visual cues in general, or *speechreading*. In addition to activities designed to enhance speech sound recognition, these classes place emphasis on the role of gestures, facial expressions, and other environmental cues that facilitate communication.

Another concept of aural rehabilitation is limited to the hearing aid evaluation and orientation process. Consistent with this orientation, another approach is to put amplification into the broader context of auditory training and to extend aural rehabilitation to include activities designed to facilitate the optimal use of residual hearing. *Auditory training* is defined as the process whereby aurally handicapped persons learn to take advantage of all acoustic cues available to them (Nicolosi, Harryman, & Kresheck, 1978). Still others view the aural rehabilitation process as providing basic information about hearing impairment and its effect on communication—a lecture series approach. Finally, there is the self-help approach. It focuses primarily on what people can do to help themselves in difficult listening situations.

In 1974 the Committee on Rehabilitative Audiology of the American Speech-Language-Hearing Association (ASHA) outlined the following components of a contemporary program:

1. Selection of an amplification system to make available as much undistorted sensory information as possible
2. Development, remediation, or conservation of receptive and expressive language abilities
3. Counseling for client and family
4. Continuing reevaluation of auditory function
5. Assessment of the effectiveness of rehabilitative procedures

TABLE 7
Goals and Components of a Comprehensive
Aural Rehabilitation Program

Prevention:	To inform the public about the nature of hearing impairment and its handicapping effects through public information programs.
Evaluation:	To assess the handicapping effects of hearing impairment for a given individual.
Remediation:	To reduce the handicapping effects of hearing impairment for a given individual.
Reevaluation:	To assess the handicapping effects of hearing impairment for a given individual following remediation activities.

Aural rehabilitation contains all of these components and more. When it is viewed narrowly, it does a partial job at best and fails miserably at worst. It follows, therefore, that an aural rehabilitation program must be designed so that it meets a wide range of the target population's needs. The program should focus on verbal communication. However, it should also center on ways in which a breakdown in the communication process impacts on other everyday activities, which should be dealt with directly, or indirectly through referral. The remainder of this monograph will discuss the essentials of a comprehensive aural rehabilitation program consistent with this point of view. Table 7 summarizes the goals and components of such a program.

Public Information Programs (Prevention)

One of the most important functions of a comprehensive aural rehabilitation program is informing the public about the nature of hearing impairment and its handicapping effects. Given that the progression of this disorder is often gradual (as in presbycusis) and that there is frequently resistance to accepting the reality of reduced hearing, the public must be provided with an opportunity to learn about the potential ramifications of hearing impairment. It is hoped that this information will come along at a time when hearing-impaired persons are just beginning to suspect that everyone else does not really mumble or talk too softly or make too much background noise, but that the problem may lie in their own inability to hear normally.

TABLE 8
Outline of a Public Information Program

Purpose:	Prevention of sustaining and increasing hearing handicap.
Process:	Community lectures, audiometric screening programs, radio and television presentations to make people aware of the handicapping effects of hearing impairment.
Content:	Hearing and Its Disorders Medical and Audiological Consultation The Adverse Effect of Poor Environmental Conditions The Value of Good Listening Habits Effective Communication Strategies Amplification as a Remedial Tool
Result:	Early identification, medical referral, and initiation of aural rehabilitation.

The public information programs can take the form of lectures and discussion groups (e.g., through social organizations or senior citizen groups) which center around hearing in general and which present the material at an elementary level. The goal is to alert the public to the numerous reasons for faulty hearing. These discussions should be designed to motivate hearing-impaired persons to seek professional help if they are experiencing difficulty. Table 8 represents an outline of such a public information program.

Evaluation

The first step in the process of planning an aural rehabilitation program for a given person is evaluation. The purpose of an evaluation is (1) to assess the handicapping effects of hearing impairment in terms of communicative efficiency and (2) to gauge the success of aural rehabilitative procedures (medical or nonmedical) in reducing these handicapping effects. This involves a thorough evaluation of both hearing impairment and hearing handicap.

Information regarding these concerns can be obtained through the administration of one or a combination of several audiometric test procedures. These procedures can be categorized into three groups: (1) threshold measures; (2) suprathreshold measures; and (3) special tests, which combine a number of psychoacoustic measures. In addition to these audiometric procedures, a num-

TABLE 9
Components of the Evaluation Process

Assessment of Hearing Impairment

Medical Referral

Assessment of Hearing Handicap

1. Communication Effect
   a. Receptive
   b. Expressive
   c. Response of auditory failure

2. Impact on the Vocational Setting

3. Impact on the Family

ber of self-report test instruments have been developed to assess another dimension of hearing handicap: a person's perceptions of the handicapping effect of the hearing impairment. The basic format of these instruments consists of presenting the hearing-impaired person with a series of questions about a potentially handicapping condition and their asking the person to judge his or her overall performance in this situation. Information of this type complements the data obtained through audiometric procedures and facilitates rehabilitative planning. For a more comprehensive discussion of these procedures see Giolas (1983). Table 9 outlines the essential components of the evaluation process.

Remediation and Reevaluation

Planning the Aural Rehabilitation Program

The evaluation process will have identified a number of potential communication difficulties experienced by the hearing-impaired person. These difficulties are generally associated with (1) the intensity of the message; (2) speech discrimination; (3) the environment, including background noise and the communication situation; and (4) response to auditory failure. An important step in planning a rehabilitative program is to discuss with the hearing-impaired person the results of the audiometric and self-report procedures in terms of communication breakdowns. This allows the hearing-impaired person to gain some insight into his or her situation and provides the clinician with the opportunity to introduce the proposed management program in terms of the person's specific hearing problems. It also provides the person with the opportunity to indicate which problems are of sufficient importance to be included early in the rehabilitation program.

At this point a specific management program is outlined. For many, this program will consist of pursuing amplification through the use of a personal hearing aid or aids. This program will include a hearing-aid evaluation and hearing-aid orientation. This phase of the aural rehabilitation program is designed to help the person make optimal use of auditory cues. In addition, a discussion regarding the handicapping effect of the hearing impairment will serve to identify problem areas and their solutions.

Optimal Use of Auditory Cues

For persons with normal hearing, the auditory modality has played the primary role in most of their mental development. Through the spoken message, complicated information has been transmitted to facilitate the acquisition of language, speech, academic, and vocational skills. The ease with which this takes place is due in large part to the multiple cues provided by verbal and nonverbal communication processes. These multiple cues are referred to by some as *redundancy cues;* they are redundant in that there are more cues than are needed to comprehend the message (Miller, 1951). The message therefore becomes predictable, and it is this predictability which makes this mode of information transmission so powerful. The primary cues contributing to the predictability of the message are in the form of physiologic, acoustic, and linguistic parameters.

It is this phenomenon of speech predictability that assists persons who acquire a hearing impairment in adulthood in compensating effectively, even though many auditory cues are diminished as a result of the disorder. With the help of amplification, many of the physiologic and acoustic cues are restored. Add to this an established internal language structure, special attention to situational cues, and a good preparatory set, and the hearing-impaired adult is often able to function satisfactorily in most listening situations. The remediation process is designed to communicate this formation to the hearing-impaired person.

Given that the major parameter of hearing impairment is reduced sensitivity as a function of frequency, the basic foundation of the remediation process is *amplification.* As more of the speech message is received, more content cues become available to the listener. Consequently, the hearing aid emerges as the

TABLE 10
Sample Hearing-Aid Orientation Program

1. Prerequisites
   (a) Hearing-aid candidacy considerations
   (b) Hearing-aid evaluation, including selection and fitting

2. Introduction to the hearing aid
   (a) How the hearing aid operates (volume switch, batteries, etc.)
   (b) Amplification through a hearing aid (advantages and limitations)

3. Assessing the effectiveness of the hearing aid (during trial period)
   (a) Observations of performance with and without the hearing aid
   (b) Evaluation of the family member or close friend
   (c) Pre- and postamplification measurements with self-report procedures
   (d) Follow-up phone calls and clinic visits
   (e) Joint meeting to make final decision

4. Handling special problems in hearing-aid adjustment
   (a) Frequent follow-up clinic visits during trial period
   (b) Participation in aural rehabilitation groups

5. Long-term follow-up
   (a) Telephone call in three months
   (b) Clinic visit in six months

Source: Giolas (1982, p. 95). Reprinted by permission.

single most important component of an aural rehabilitation program for this population.

The appropriate use of amplification is so important to a remediation program that the ultimate effectiveness of the program is dependent upon successful hearing-aid use. Clinicians know of too many hearing-impaired persons who are not wearing their hearing aids at all or who are using them improperly. This is primarily a function of poor management. A carefully designed program of hearing-aid orientation must be an integral part of an aural rehabilitation program. The goal of such a program should be to help hearing-impaired persons receive optimal benefit from their personal hearing aid. A sample hearing-aid orientation program is outlined in Table 10. This program assumes a carefully conducted hearing-aid evaluation and fitting procedure by a clinical audiologist.

A well-planned hearing-aid orientation program will ordinarily be sufficient to start the postlingually hearing-impaired person on the road to making optimal use of his or her residual hearing through the use of amplification. However, some suggest that more extensive auditory training can be helpful. McCarthy and Alpiner (1982) list the following goals of auditory training: (1) recognition of those sounds which are incorrectly discriminated; (2) pre– and post–hearing-aid orientation, including adjustment to amplification; and (3) improvement of tolerance levels. McCarthy and Alpiner discuss a number of auditory training activities that can be used in a group or individual setting. They stress, however, that a thorough evaluation of the person's auditory training needs must precede any management program.

Communication Strategies

Optimal use of residual hearing through the successful use of a hearing aid will not completely eliminate all auditory failure. Auditory failure occurs as a result of uncorrectable distortion of the spoken message due to the organic hearing impairment and adverse environmental conditions. It becomes the responsibility of the hearing-impaired person to develop strategies to compensate for such difficulties. These strategies can be grouped into three categories: (1) use of visual and situational cues; (2) manipulation of the physical environment; and (3) constructive response to auditory failure. Each of these is discussed in this section.

These communication strategies are best introduced and developed in a group setting, where discussion and role playing can be used to demonstrate the principles involved. These aural rehabilitative groups provide a dynamic setting in which interaction between peers (hearing-impaired persons), family members, and the group leader (the audiologist) generates productive discussions and, most important, solutions to communication problems. The emphasis placed on each category of communication strategies will vary with the group members' needs. Table 11 outlines the purpose and format of these groups. As the table suggests, activities centering on the optimal use of auditory cues as described earlier are often included as part of the group activities.

One of the more productive compensatory communication strategies used in difficult listening situations is increased reliance on the nonverbal cues inherent in all communication settings. This strategy is based on the assumption that lip movements, facial expressions, gestures, and situational cues offer meaningful supplementary information regarding the content of the conversation. Coupled with the amplified auditory cues provided by the hearing aid, the visual cues accompanying oral communication can enhance the process of decoding the auditory message. Consequently, group activities are conducted to develop

TABLE 11
Aural Rehabilitation Groups

Purpose:	To provide supportive and substantive help to persons having communication problems associated with hearing impairment.
Goal:	To analyze auditory failures and to develop concrete behaviors that result in improved communication.
Process:	The group process, with the audiologist serving as the group leader.
Rationale:	The group process provides a setting in which there is considerable exchange of information, mutual support, and validation of communication problems and solutions.
Format:	Role of the Group Leader

Facilitator of discussion
A good listener
Expert on hearing and its disorders

Session Structure

Presentation of content (through films, lectures, etc.)
Supervised group discussion
Communication strategies activities
Home assignments

Group Members

Hearing-impaired persons
Close friends or family members with whom communication is
     important and frequent

Group Activities

Optimal use of auditory cues
Optimal use of visual cues
Manipulation of environment
Response to auditory failure

a greater awareness of the value of using nonauditory cues. This heightened awareness is not difficult to develop and becomes more or less natural as its value is experienced.

Several activities are conducted to illustrate the general advantages of using nonverbal cues. Initially, activities are designed to highlight the value of visual cues in general (i.e., facial expressions, gestures, and situational cues). Later, activities centering around lipreading per se are conducted to illustrate the supplementary role of this type of visual cue. Some prefer the term speechreading to lipreading. Speech reading is thought to be a comprehensive term suggesting the use of a broader scope of visual cues in addition to just lip movements. Speechreading has merit and the general acceptance of professionals; however, lipreading is still the more natural term for the lay person. It is important that aural rehabilitation programs include emphasis on both the use of visual cues in general (speechreading) as well as the specific cues derived from lip movements (lipreading).

In a comprehensive program, care is taken to discuss the limitations of lipreading as an information channel for verbal messages. The advantages and limitations of lipreading are pointed out, with examples or activities illustrating each of them. While most persons with a postlingual hearing impairment will seldom need to depend upon lipreading exclusively, clues obtained from watching the lips are obviously available. Many potential acoustic confusions can be avoided by a combination of contextual and visual cues. For example, the acoustically similar verbal requests "Pass the cheese" and "Pass the peas" could cause confusion. Contextual cues would not help differentiate between *cheese* and *peas,* but visual cues would. Helping people become aware of the probability of this type of confusion will go a long way toward motivating them to watch the speaker. On the other hand, the limitations of depending upon lipreading alone are best illustrated by turning down the sound of the television set and suddenly noticing how little can be gleaned from the silent lip movements on the screen. Even with a familiar program that one has been watching and listening to for quite a while, the words and phrases escape one.

The group leader should point out that very few people with a postlingual hearing impairment are sufficiently impaired to require total dependence on visual cues alone and that is is extremely difficult (if not impossible) to carry on an extensive discussion with just lipreading alone, since only one thired of the sounds are visible. To carry on a lengthy conversation requires additional visual and auditory cues.

Consistent with the goal of educating both hearing-impaired persons and their families in the rehabilitation process, all group members are invited to participate in these activities at one time or another. The value of activities of this type lies in the discussions that follow. Time is allowed for the participants to analyze their failure and/or success with the lipreading activities. How do they approach it? Do they give up when they have not understood the first few words, or do they keep trying to look for contextual cues? Do they state what they thought was said and ask for confirmation? Do they ask for the whole sentence to be repeated? Do they take a guess? All of these strategies and others are typically displayed in a lipreading activity. They are also responses common to all communication settings. Some are effective, and others are counterproductive and should not be used. The lipreading activity provides a real-life situation in which to demonstrate the preferred communication strategies. With simple modifications of this basic lipreading activity, additional communication strategies of general applicability can be introduced and practiced. Guidelines for lipreading activities developed by Giolas (1982) as well as Erickson's (1974) excellent suggestions for improving speechreading effectiveness are recommended.

Thus, lipreading activities provide a fine opportunity to present communication strategies that are available to the hearing-impaired adult. Little or no attention is paid to whether there is improvement in lipreading per se but rather improvement in the approach to deciphering the auditory-visual code. No formal lipreading tests are administered. This would place too much emphasis on lipreading and would be inconsistent with the group's goal of placing lipreading in a broader context. The assessment of visual cues obtained during the evaluation stage of the aural rehabilitation program is used to identify general areas to be stressed in the group sessions.

The setting in which the communication act takes place plays an important role in how well a person will hear and understand what is being said. This is especially true for the hearing-impaired person whose *redundancy* cues have been reduced by the hearing impairment. Consequently, environmental conditions such as background noise, lighting, number of people talking, and distance from the speaker can contribute to auditory failure. Whenever possible, these conditions should be optimized to improve communication efficiency. Giolas (1982) outlined the following guidelines to help a hearing-impaired person improve communication settings:

1. Create a relatively noise-free environment. This includes requesting that background music be turned down or off, closing the door to minimize external noise, and meeting with others in rooms with good acoustics.
2. Secure the most advantageous position relative to the speaker(s). For public events (meetings, hearings, lectures, church services, etc.), arrive early so that you can sit near the front and in a position to see all speakers.
3. At informal gatherings limit the number of speakers whom you engage in conversation at one time. One-to-one conversations are easier than group conversations.

4. Correct poor lighting conditions in order to facilitate the use of all nonverbal cues. Dimly lit restaurants are prime examples of poor lighting conditions. There are often tables that are better lighted than others.
5. Encourage the use of public-address systems when they are available.

The consequences of not having heard and/or understood what was said are often the result of the person's response to the particular auditory failure. If the person does something to correct the situation, the consequences are mostly negated. For example, when a person misses a point being made and asks for it to be repeated, the speaker usually does this so that the information is received correctly by the hearing-impaired person, and the conversation continues. In this example, no sustaining communication breakdown occurred because it was corrected immediately. A problem occurs only when an auditory failure goes unchecked, leading to subsequent misunderstandings of what was said. Therefore, hearing-impaired persons must develop a repertoire of successful responses to auditory failure, such as those suggested by Giolas (1982):

1. When you are aware that you missed something that was said, ask for it to be repeated. Repeat the portions you heard to facilitate the flow of the conversation.
2. If someone is talking unusually softly, adjust your hearing aid to hear that person better.
3. Whenever possible, inform the speaker that you have a hearing impairment and suggest what he or she can do to help you understand.
4. Avoid pretending you understood what was said. It will only confuse things later.
5. If you cannot interrupt the speaker, ask someone near you to fill you in on what you did not hear.
6. Even though you feel you are missing a lot, keep trying to follow the discussion. Some nonverbal or situational cues will often emerge to get you back on the track.
7. Ask someone near you to alert you to changes in the topic of conversation.

Table 12 summarizes the group activities typically included in a standard aural rehabilitation group program.

Groups vs. Individual Sessions

It is not always possible or appropriate to conduct aural rehabilitation in a group setting. Often a person's personal schedule conflicts with the time of the group meetings. Sometimes the person's hearing loss is sufficiently severe so as to make participation in group discussion difficult. Still others might prefer to meet

TABLE 12
Examples of Group Activities Included
in Aural Rehabilitation Groups

Optimal Use of Auditory Cues

    Amplification considerations
    Hearing-aid orientation

Communication Strategies

    Optimal use of visual cues
      Role of redundancy
      Role of visual cues in general
      Role of lipreading
        Contribute to understanding conversational speech
        Limitations
        Use of lipreading activities to develop a general approach to communication
        breakdowns

    Manipulation of environment
    Response to auditory failure

individually with the audiologist until they become more comfortable with their hearing impairment. Often administrative conditions within the clinical setting dictate that aural rehabilitation be conducted on an individual basis. Whether the rehabilitative process is conducted individually or within a group, the goal and principles are identical. In both situations, the clinician is interested in helping persons with a hearing impairment develop effective compensatory communication strategies. The major difference between the two situations lies in the number of people involved in helping to identify the solutions. In the individual format the discussion takes place between two people (or three if the spouse can be included) rather than among several, as in the group format. The group discussion process is still used.

Individual sessions are often conducted as part of the group format. These sessions provide an opportunity to discuss issues or communication strategies specific to the person's needs. Finally, individual sessions are conducted when more personal issues associated with hearing impairment need to be discussed.

An obvious example of persons with whom individual sessions work quite effectively are persons with a unilateral hearing impairment. As indicated earlier, persons with unilateral hearing exhibit communication problems and have negative feelings about their impairment and the situations in which they experience communication difficulty. One good ear does not afford normal hearing for all practical purposes.

While persons with unilateral hearing do not require the extensive aural rehabilitation suggested for the bilaterally hearing-impaired adult, it should be pointed out that they will most likely have difficulty localizing the direction from which sound is coming and understanding speech when the talker is located on the side of the poor ear or when there is background noise in the listening environment. Assuming the hearing impairment is medically irreversible, the goals of rehabilitation are twofold: (1) to reduce negative emotions related to the hearing impairment and (2) to develop more effective actions in response to adverse listening situations.

The use of amplification with persons having unilateral hearing impairment has already been suggested by Harford and Barry (1965) and Harford and Dodds (1966). In instances where amplification is appropriate, hearing-aid orientation will also be needed, geared of course to the special problems associated with unilateral hearing.

It should be pointed out that special evaluation procedures have not been developed to systematically assess the communication problems experienced by a given person with a unilateral hearing impairment. The clinician must therefore improvise, using procedures such as those developed for the bilaterally hearing-impaired person.

Another group of persons for whom individual work is most appropriate and productive is persons with a sudden hearing impairment. Generally, the problems associated with a sudden severe bilateral hearing impairment are similar to the problems exhibited by a person with gradual hearing impairment. However, they are complicated by the sudden onset and by the severity of the loss. The initial psychological impact of such a loss is so great that resistance to aural rehabilitation is often marked. The impact of a sudden bilateral severe hearing impairment is best understood in terms of Ramsdell's three psychological levels of hearing (primitive, signal or warning, and symbolic), which were discussed earlier.

The rehabilitative process for the person with a sudden hearing impairment varies. It is determined by a number of factors, including the extent and type of the hearing impairment; the degree to which the person is visually oriented; the person's work situation; the person's general lifestyle and basic approach to personal problems; and the family's understanding of the problem and overall support.

Initially, considerable time is spent talking with the hearing-impaired person and his or her family. All persons involved are provided with the opportunity to ask questions about the status of the individual's hearing, the cause of the impairment, the management plan, and the prognosis for improvement. Throughout this discussion the audiologist strives to play a supportive role. Remedial activities are initiated as soon as possible to provide the person and his or her family with a sense of success and progress. At the same time, the plan should be sufficiently flexible to allow for digression when hearing-impaired persons wish to pursue questions about why they feel as they do, what the future holds for them, and what concerns they may have about their hearing. Throughout this management program, the audiologist is always on the lookout for signs pointing to a psychological referral.

Whenever possible, at least one family member or close friend should be included in most management sessions. This will provide both parties with an opportunity to work on new communication patterns under the supervision of the audiologist. It will also help the person with normal hearing develop a better understanding of the hearing-impaired person's communication situation.

The evaluation procedures described earlier may be used with this population if their administration and use are modified to meet the adjustment status of the person being treated. The evaluation procedure is usually spread out over more time so as to allow remediation to be initiated earlier than is needed with other types of hearing impairments.

Amplification is tried as soon as possible. Its success depends on a variety of factors, including the severity of the loss, its etiology, and the person's willingness to give the hearing aid a fair trial. The trial period is accompanied by intensive hearing-aid orientation activities similar to those described earlier. The hearing-impaired person is helped to understand that even though the hearing aid does not restore speech to its previous clarity, coupled with visual and situational cues it can help improve communication efficiency. For some people, it will contribute more to reestablishing the primitive and signal-warning levels of hearing than the symbolic level.

The activities designed to foster increased use of visual cues that were described earlier are most important and productive with this population. Vision symbolizes a significant safety factor and represents a major approach to compensating for the hearing impairment. Most importantly, it provides a vehicle through which to present communication strategies applicable to all hearing-impaired persons. Consequently, intensive work on the use of visual cues (including speechreading) comprises a major part of the management program. Individual as well as small-group (one or two family members) sessions become the standard management format for these activities.

The Elderly

The aural rehabilitation groups described in this monograph are quite appropriate for the elderly person. In many ways, common denominators like age, general interests, adjustment patterns, and stage of life often make a group approach more effective with elderly persons then with more heterogenous groups. Because the aging process in general has often created a general reduction in responsiveness to verbal messages, it is sometimes advisable to reduce the group size. This in turn will reduce the potential number of verbal exchanges and make it easier for the group members to follow the group activities. If the meetings can be held in familiar settings, with members who regularly interact and at a convenient time, aural rehabilitation groups can be the most rewarding approach to helping the older person with a hearing problem. As with all groups, the group leader takes care to select activities commensurate with the maturity and experiences of the members. If a group of people have lived in the geographic area for many years, discussions of familiar subjects (e.g., how things used to be and the history of old landmarks, etc.) provide an abundance of materials to implement the communication strategy activities described earlier. In that many elderly people are extremely dependent on family members or close friends for social outlets and transportation, it is especially important to include family and friends in the group activities. This will facilitate improvement in all aspects of these personal relationships.

The Educational Setting

More and more colleges and universities are opening their doors to the hearing-impaired student. The era of mainstreaming the hearing-handicapped person is here, and the role of the university audiology clinic is clear. It should become the home base for hearing-impaired students in the college or university setting. It should work closely with the student and school personnel to determine the nature of supportive services needed by the hearing-impaired student. This will involve a careful evaluation of the student's hearing handicap, with special consideration given to the student's educational listening situation and appropriate personal and education amplification needs. More specifically, the clinic should help the student explore the feasibility of using a radio frequency (FM) amplification unit in the classroom.

Most universities have an office of services for the handicapped. The hearing-impaired person should be put in touch with such an office. These offices are often able to provide services such as tutoring, oral or manual interpreting, a note-taker, special arrangements for test-taking, and others. They also often work very closely with the state vocational rehabilitation office and can put the hearing-impaired student in touch with this agency.

Most importantly, hearing-impaired students should view the university audiology clinic as a resource center where they can secure the appropriate advice and support when special problems arise during their college stay. Many times, these students can serve as role models for parents and aural rehabilitation groups attending the clinic. This not only helps the service program but gives hearing-impaired students an opportunity to share their understanding of the hearing handicap and communication strategies.

The nature and extent of the student's involvement will depend on the severity of the hearing loss. While the clinic should make itself available to all hearing-impaired students, it is most likely the severely hearing-impaired students will need the most help. There is much that can be done to help them, and many times the degree to which the university audiology clinic becomes involved with the student may well determine the success of the student's educational experience.

TABLE 13
The Remediation Process

Purpose
  To reduce the handicapping effects of hearing impairment, with special emphasis on communication performance (i.e., component of the communication process).

Issues for Consideration
  Nature of Hearing Impairment
    Medical and Audiological Evaluations
  Nature of Hearing Handicap
    Audiological Evaluation
  Appropriate Referral(s)
    Medical, Counseling, etc.
  Amplification Needs
    Hearing Aid(s), Assistive Devices, etc.
  Compensatory Communication Strategy Needs
    Speechreading, Manipulation of the Environment, etc.

Management Program
  Discussion of test results and observations with hearing-impaired person and family

  Work individually with hearing-impaired person on amplification and compensatory communication strategy needs

  If needed, include in an aural rehabilitation group

Summary

A comprehensive aural rehabilitation program for persons who acquired a hearing impairment as an adult has been discussed. The major components of such a program consist of (1) public information prevention, (2) evaluation, (3) remediation, and (4) reevaluation. The service delivery sequence outlined includes (1) medical and audiological evaluation, (2) amplification considerations, and (3) a program of communication strategies. For the most part, this remediation process facilitates the indentification of persons' special aural rehabilitation needs and management program. The rehabilitative process consists of demonstrating the need for active and aggressive listening and offering practice in how to accomplish this goal. Table 13 represents an outline of the remediation process.

References

Alpiner, J. G. (1979). Psychological and social aspects of aging as related to hearing rehabilitation of elderly clients. In M. Henoch (Ed.), *Aural rehabilitation for the elderly* (pp. 169–184). New York: Grune & Stratton.

American National Standards Institute. (1970). *Specifications for audiometers* (ANSI 53.6–1969). New York: American National Standards Institute.

American Speech and Hearing Association, Committee on Rehabilitative Audiology. (1974). The audiologist: Responsibilities in the habilitation of the auditorily handicapped. *ASHA, 16* (2), 68–70.

Binnie, C. A. (1973). Bisensory articulation functions for normal hearing and sensorineural hearing loss patients. *Journal of the Academy of Rehabilitative Audiology, 6,* 43–53.

Crum, M. A., & Tillman, T. W. (1973). *Effects of speaker-to-noise distance upon speech intelligibility in reverberation and noise.* Paper presented at a meeting of the American Speech and Hearing Association, Detroit, MI.

Davis, H., & Silverman, S. R. (1978). *Hearing and deafness* (4th ed.). New York: Holt, Rinehart & Winston.

Erikson, J. G. (1978). *Speech reading: An aid to communication.* Danville, IL: Interstate Printers & Publishers.

Fein, D. J. (1983). Projections of speech and hearing impairments to 2050. *ASHA, 25*(11), 31.

Flanagan, J. C. (1954). The critical incident technique. *Psychological Bulletin, 51,* 351–358.

Fleming, M. (1972). A total approach to communication therapy. *Journal of the Academy of Rehabilitative Audiology, 5,* 28–31.

Gaeth, J. (1948). *A study of phonemic regression associated with hearing loss.* Unpublished doctoral dissertation, Northwestern University, Chicago.

Giolas, T. G. (1982). *Hearing-handicapped adults.* Englewood Cliffs, NJ: Prentice-Hall.

Giolas, T. G. (1983). The self-assessment approach in audiology: State of the art. *Audiology, 8*(11), 157–171.

Giolas, T. G., & Wark, D. J. (1967). Communication problems associated with unilateral hearing loss. *Journal of Speech and Hearing Disorders, 32*(4), 336–342.

Glorig, A., Wheeler, D., Quiggle, R., Grings, W., & Summerfield, A. (1957). *1954 Wisconsin State Fair hearing survey.* American Academy of Opthalmology and Otolaryngology Monograph. Washington, DC: American Academy of Opthalmology and Otolaryngolgy.

Harford, E., & Barry, J. (1965). A rehabilitative approach to the problem of unilateral hearing impairment: Contralateral routing of signal (CROS). *Journal of Speech and Hearing Disorders, 30,* 121–138.

Harford, E., & Dodds, B. (1966). The clinical application of CROS. *Archives of Otolaryngology, 83,* 455–464.

Hull, R. H. (1977). *Hearing impairment among aging persons.* Lincoln, NE: Cliffs Notes.

Lipscomb, D. M. (1970). Noise in the environment: The problem. *Maco Audiological Library Series, 8*(1), 1–6.

Martin, F. N. (1981). *Introduction to audiology* (2nd ed.). Englewood Cliffs, NJ: Prentice-Hall.

McCarthy, P. A., & Alpiner, J. G. (1978). The remediation process. In J.G. Alpiner (Ed.), *Handbook of adult rehabilitative audiology* (2nd ed., pp. 99–136). Baltimore: Willliams & Wilkins.

Miller, G. A. (1951). *Language and communication.* New York: McGraw-Hill.

Nabelek, A. K., & Pickett, J. M. (1947a). Reception of consonants in a classroom as affected by monaural and binaural listening, noise reverberation and hearing aids. *Journal of the Acoustical Society of America, 56,* 628–639.

Nabelek, A. K., & Pickett, J. M. (1947b). Monaural and binaural speech perception through hearing aids under noise and reverberation with normal and hearing-impaired listeners. *Journal of Speech and Hearing Research, 17,* 724–739.

National Center for Health Statistics. (1982). *Unpublished data from 1980 National Health Interview Survey.* Washington, DC: National Center for Health Statistics.

Nett, E. M., Doerfler, L. G., & Matthews, J. (1960). *The relationship between audiological measures and handicap.* Unpublished manuscript. Vocational Rehabilitation Adminstration, Project No. 167. Washington, DC: Department of Education, Office of Special Education.

Nicolosi, L., Harryman, E., & Kresheck, J. (1978). *Terminology of communication disorder.* Baltimore: Williams & Wilkins.

Noble, W. G. (1978). *Assessment of the hearing impaired: A critique and a new method.* New York: Academic Press.

O'Neill, J. J., & Oyer, H. J. (1961). *Visual communication for the hard of hearing.* Englewood Cliffs, NJ: Prentice-Hall.

Owens, E., Benedict, M., & Schubert, E. D. (1972). Consonant phonemic errors associated with pure-tone configurations and certain kinds of hearing impairment. *Journal of Speech and Hearing Research, 15,* 308–322.

Owens, E., & Fujikawa, S. (1980). The H.P.I. and hearing aid use in profound hearing loss. *Journal of Speech and Hearing Disorders, 23,* 473–479.

Owens, E., & Schubert, E. D. (1968a). The development of consonant items for speech discrimination testing. *Journal of Speech and Hearing Research, 11,* 656–667.

Owens, E., Talbott, C. B., & Schubert, E. D. (1968b). Vowel discrimination of hearing-impaired listeners. *Journal of Speech and Hearing Research, 11,* 649–655.

Punch, J. (1983). The prevalence of hearing impairment. *ASHA, 24*(4), 27.

Ramsdell, O. A. (1978). The psychology of the hard-of-hearing and the deafened adult. In H. Davis & S. R. Silverman (Eds.), *Hearing and deafness* (4th ed., pp. 499–510). New York: Holt, Rinehart & Winston.

Ross, M. (1978). Classroom acoustics and speech intelligibility. In J. Katz (Ed.), *Handbook of clinical audiology* (pp. 469–478). Baltimore: Williams & Wilkins.

Rousey, C. (1971). Psychological reactions to hearing loss. *Journal of Speech and Hearing Disorders, 36,* 382–389.

Shontz, F. C. (1967). Reactions to crisis. *Volta Review, 69,* 405–411.

Shostrom, E. L. (1967). *Man the manipulator.* Nashville, TN: Abingdon Press.

Tillman, T. W., Carhart, R., & Olsen, W. O. (1974). Hearing aid efficiency in a competing speech situation. *Journal of Speech and Hearing Research, 13,* 789–811.

Thomas G. Giolas is Professor of Audiology in the Department of Communication Sciences at the University of Connecticut. He also serves as the acting director of the University of Connecticut Research Foundation. He is the author of *Hearing-Handicapped Adults*, co-author (with Kenneth Randolph) of *Basic Audiometry, Including Impedance Measurement*, and co-editor (with Mark Ross) of *Auditory Management of Hearing-Impaired Children*. He is also the author of numerous chapters, articles, and conference papers in his field. Dr. Giolas is a Fellow of the American Speech-Language-Hearing Association of America. He is a previous editorial consultant for the *Journal of Speech and Hearing Disorders* and is currently serving in that capacity for the *Journal of the Academy of Rehabilitative Audiology*.